Sodium Counter Book

A Beginner's Quick Start Guide to Counting Sodium, With a
Sodium Food List and Low Sodium Sample Recipes

SODIUM COUNTER BOOK

Disclaimer

By reading this disclaimer, you are accepting the terms of the disclaimer in full. If you disagree with this disclaimer, please do not read the guide.

All of the content within this guide is provided for informational and educational purposes only, and should not be accepted as independent medical or other professional advice. The author is not a doctor, physician, nurse, mental health provider, or registered nutritionist/dietician. Therefore, using and reading this guide does not establish any form of a physician-patient relationship.

Always consult with a physician or another qualified health provider with any issues or questions you might have regarding any sort of medical condition. Do not ever disregard any qualified professional medical advice or delay seeking that advice because of anything you have read in this guide. The information in this guide is not intended to be any sort of medical advice and should not be used in lieu of any medical advice by a licensed and qualified medical professional.

The information in this guide has been compiled from a variety of known sources. However, the author cannot attest to or guarantee the accuracy of each source and thus should not be held liable for any errors or omissions.

You acknowledge that the publisher of this guide will not be held liable for any loss or damage of any kind incurred as a result of this guide or the reliance on any information provided within this guide. You acknowledge and agree that you assume all risk and responsibility for any action you undertake in response to the information in this guide.

Using this guide does not guarantee any particular result (e.g., weight loss or a cure). By reading this guide, you acknowledge that there are no guarantees to any specific outcome or results you can expect.

All product names, diet plans, or names used in this guide are for identification purposes only and are the property of their respective owners. The use of these names does not imply endorsement. All other trademarks cited herein are the property of their respective owners.

Where applicable, this guide is not intended to be a substitute for the original work of this diet plan and is, at most, a supplement to the original work for this diet plan and never a direct substitute. This guide is a personal expression of the facts of that diet plan.

Where applicable, persons shown in the cover images are stock photography models and the publisher has obtained the rights to use the images through license agreements with third-party stock image companies.

Introduction

Did you know that the recommended sodium intake by the American Heart Association (AHA) should not exceed 1,500 milligrams per day? However, most people actually consume more than twice that number—about 3,400 milligrams.

According to research, at least 9 out of 10 people exceed the dietary limit for sodium intake. What is shocking is that the majority of the sodium we consume comes directly from food processing. You will discover that even foods that may not taste salty are loaded with high quantities of sodium.

Sodium is a mineral needed by the body to function well. It helps maintain fluid balance, regulate nerves and muscles, and control blood volume and pressure, to say the least. However, too much of anything isn't always a good thing. That's why there are regulations as to how much is recommended for daily consumption according to experts. Excessive sodium consumption may result in problems with heart and blood pressure. This is why people with kidney diseases and high blood pressure are strictly advised to watch their sodium consumption.

This guide is designed to give you some basic information about sodium and then provide you with a list of recommended food items with low sodium content. Sample recipes are also offered at the end.

In this guide, you will learn:

• Reasons why too much sodium is bad for your health
• How to count sodium
• Foods high in sodium
• Foods low in sodium
• Sodium food list and their sodium content

So, are you trying to ditch salt from your diet? Well, this guide is precisely what you need! Read on and find out more.

All About Sodium

Sodium is a mineral your body needs to function, but too much can lead to high blood pressure and other problems. It's a major electrolyte, which means it helps maintain fluid balance in the body, conduct nerve impulses, and promote muscle contraction, including your heart. Thus, maintaining balanced sodium levels is critical for healthy bodily function.

Because sodium affects the fluid balance in the body, it also affects
blood pressure. This means that if you consume high quantities of sodium in your diet, you are likely to have high blood pressure.

Perhaps you are wondering how it happens. Simple. Water goes to where sodium is. In that case, if the sodium concentration is high in the blood, it results in increased water retention, which causes an increase in pressure in the blood vessels.

At first, high blood pressure may not be much of a problem. However, it damages the blood vessel walls with time, which leads to a cascade of events that ultimately cause cardiovascular complications such as stroke or heart failure.

For most healthy people, the body needs a small amount every day, around 500mg. However, watching how much sodium you have is essential because having too much can lead to health problems—including high blood pressure and kidney disease—over time. Sodium levels are measured in milligrams per liter (mg/L) of blood serum. The Dietary Guidelines for Americans recommend keeping sodium intake below 2,300 mg/day. ALA, as mentioned earlier, recommends an even lower bar, strictly 1,500 mg/day.

A milligram or mg is simply 1/1,000 of a gram (g). A liter is ~ 1 quart. To help you visualize, 1 liter = 10.8 ounces (oz), and therefore 1,000 milligrams = 0.62 oz or, roughly, 3/4 of a teaspoon of salt.

Suppose you have chronic kidney disease, heart problems, or another health condition that requires limiting sodium intake. In that case, it's essential to follow the specific guidelines set for your health situation.

Sodium is found naturally in some foods, but most of the time, it's added during processing or preparing food, for example, canned vegetables. Thus, knowing which foods are high in sodium can help you plan for healthy meals throughout the week. It will also be helpful if you're looking into one of our recipes that calls for ingredients like canned vegetables or soups.

Some people are less sensitive to sodium, while others are not. People who are less susceptible to sodium tend to consume more sodium without necessarily triggering an increase in their blood pressure. This sensitivity is often linked to hereditary factors, but it is hard to know where you stand without testing it. Therefore, the most reasonable thing to do is be mindful of how much sodium you consume in your diet every day. Don't go overboard with your consumption!

Problems with Too Much Sodium

Over time, too much sodium can lead to health issues like high blood pressure, also called hypertension. It's estimated that 1 in 3 adults has high blood pressure. You can have lower blood pressure just by making some changes to your diet and getting more exercise every day, which may translate into a reduced risk of heart disease, stroke, kidney disease, eye problems, and other health conditions.

Reducing sodium does not mean cutting out all salt (sodium chloride). Instead, it is about replacing high-sodium foods with low-sodium alternatives or finding ways to prepare favorite foods in new ways by adding fresh ingredients or using alternate cooking methods like grilling instead of frying. Thus, eating smaller amounts of certain foods—for example, deli meat—or using spices and flavors to make dishes more interesting despite lessening or not using salt at all.

Some of the health conditions that too much sodium can aggravate are as follows:

High blood pressure

High blood pressure is often called the "silent killer" because it has no symptoms, so you may not know you have it. If your blood pressure is consistently high, it puts added stress on your heart. You are then at serious risk for heart disease or stroke.

It is typically diagnosed with a blood pressure test. Ask your doctor what your blood pressure numbers should be and which category you fit in (normal, prehypertension, or hypertension).

This is generally treated with lifestyle changes, medication, or both. Treating high blood pressure may involve making wise choices about the foods that contain sodium, getting active, and exercising more. If you smoke cigarettes or use chewing tobacco, quitting will benefit nearly every organ in your body.

Heart disease
This is the leading cause of death for men and women in the United States. It can lead to sudden cardiac arrest, which can be fatal, or coronary heart disease (CHD), which includes conditions such as angina and coronary artery disease.

Heart failure
When your heart can't pump enough blood to meet your body's needs, your heart fails to function. If the problem is severe, fluid may back up in your lungs and leave you short of breath, or fluid may build up in other parts of your body, such as your ankles and legs.

Kidney disease
Chronic kidney disease (CKD) happens when your kidneys are damaged and can't filter waste and fluids from the blood like they usually do. Your kidneys play a vital role: toxins can build to dangerous levels in your body without healthy kidneys and cause severe damage, including death. If you have CKD, dialysis treatments help eliminate wastes that would otherwise build up in your system.

Not everyone who has high blood pressure, heart disease, or kidney disease needs to limit sodium in their diet. However, many people would benefit from doing so because they could lower their risk of developing these conditions. They also might reduce the chances of having a stroke or other cardiovascular diseases.

Sodium is harmful when consumed in excess amounts. It can raise blood pressure and increase water retention, ultimately leading to high-risk health issues such as heart disease, obesity, and kidney problems. Some individuals are more sensitive to the impacts of salt than others who may require less dietary sodium intake while still reaping its benefits. This Sodium Counter Guide references how much sodium is contained in certain foods that you eat throughout the day while providing low-sodium versions of popular recipes so you can enjoy a variety of foods without sacrificing your health.

How to Count Sodium

Many food labels have a Nutrition Facts section, which lists how much sodium is in the product. Here's what to look for on the label:

The "Sodium or salt" line indicates how many milligrams of sodium is in one serving of the product. For example, if there is about 220 mg of sodium in each serving, it appears like this: 220mg (of sodium) per serving.

The "% Daily Value (DV)" line shows how much one serving contributes to your total daily limit based on an average 2000-calorie diet. It also includes information about the % daily value of other nutrients, such as fat and cholesterol.

This example shows that one serving provides 10% of your daily limit for sodium—meaning you can eat ~22 servings and still stay below the recommended daily limit for sodium (2300 mg).

The following line (in this case, it says "Not a significant source of dietary fiber") indicates what is in the product.

Reviewing food labels should also include how much sodium is in each ingredient used to make the product. For example, here's the list of ingredients for taco seasoning:

On this label, 2 tbsp. (or around 21 g) would contribute 1470 mg to the total sodium content present in the entire package. By reading labels carefully, consumers can avoid foods high in sodium.

While it is not healthy to consume high sodium in the diet, there are various ways you can counter the amounts. The trick is to modify your diet to dilute the sodium concentration in the blood. Here's how:

Increase your Potassium intake
Did you know that sodium and potassium have complementary functions in the human body?

Well, now you know!

While sodium promotes water retention and increases blood pressure, potassium does the opposite—flushes out excess fluid from the blood and lowers blood pressure. Therefore, if your sodium intake is abnormally high, increasing your potassium intake goes a long way in helping you achieve balance.

The recommended daily dietary intake of potassium is 4.7 grams. Unfortunately, most people don't even reach the 50% mark. One large banana gives you at least 400 mg of potassium. In that case, you need to consume lots of foods loaded with potassium to counter your sodium levels. Some potassium-rich foods include; spinach, banana, dried fruit, lima beans, and fish. Ensuring that you consume these foods across meals will give your body all the daily potassium it needs, countering sodium intake.

Drink plenty of water

As mentioned earlier, when your sodium intake is too high, the body will try to dilute the salt by retaining as much water as possible—bloating. By increasing your water intake, the body can cut the excess sodium and eliminate the bloating feeling.

In case you are wondering about how much water you should consume, this depends on your activity levels. If you burn at least 2,000 calories daily, you need to consume at least two liters. However, if you are an athlete, you need at least four times the amount.

Increase your physical activity
Working out has been shown to play a vital role in helping the body get rid of excess sodium from the blood. When you exercise, the body loses water and salts in the form of sweat. That said, maintaining good hydration is critical in ensuring that your body functions well.

Take note, though rare, that consuming too much water may cause the sodium levels to be too low. Therefore, when exercising under hot conditions where sweating is significantly increased, you must consume some salts while ensuring that you keep your body well hydrated.

Ditch the salt shaker

When cooking, it is easy to introduce high sodium in the food if you are not mindful. However, cooking is one of the best ways to control how much sodium you consume. Some of the tricks that will lower your sodium intake during cooking include;

- Holding the salt and instead of using spices and herbs to season food. Some herbs you can use include basil, lemon zest, rosemary, ginger, garlic, black pepper, cayenne pepper, paprika, and others.
- Lowering the amount of baking powder used in baking because of its high sodium content.
- Rinsing veggies and canned beans under cold water to wash away the sodium before cooking.
- Marinating with vinegar and citrus juices instead of salts.

This does not mean that your food will taste bland!

When you lower the amount of salt used in cooking, you can taste the natural flavors in your food. With time, your taste buds will gradually adjust to less salt, and it soon becomes your preference.

Foods High in Sodium

Most of the sodium you consume comes from eating processed foods and restaurant meals. There are a few naturally-occurring food sources where significant amounts can be found (like celery and milk). Still, those aren't the primary contributors to your overall intake for the most part. Instead, it's generally those prepared or packaged items that bring up your daily sodium levels.

Here is a quick list for reference:
• Pretzels
• Cold cuts
• Soup
• Packaged dinners and side dishes
• Chicken flavored ramen or soup (without vegetables)
• Canned beans/vegetables (look for low sodium varieties if you need to limit sodium intake)
• Macaroni and cheese
• Salted nuts
• Canned soups
• Meatloaves
• Hot dogs
• Salsa
• Ketchup or catsup (look for low sodium options)
• Other sauces like soy sauce, teriyaki sauce, and steak sauce (use them sparingly).

As you can see, most of the foods here are highly processed or prepared. In general, it's much easier to cut these kinds of foods from your diet as much as possible. Look for healthier alternatives, such as fresh vegetables and fruits, legumes/beans, whole grains, and lean protein sources like dairy, eggs, fish, and meat without the skin.

Foods Low in Sodium

Now that you know which foods to avoid or limit, it's also essential to know which foods are better for your health and don't contribute as much sodium.

Here is a list of low-sodium options:

- Fresh vegetables
  - Asparagus
  - Broccoli
  - Cucumbers
  - Spinach
  - Garlic
  - Eggplant
  - Green beans
  - Squash

These veggies are packed with nutrients that play a critical role in lowering blood cholesterol levels and pressure. You boost your heart health by upping your vegetable intake, especially leafy greens.

Also, when prepping your veggies, don't overcook them lest they lose their nutrients in the process. The best cooking methods are steaming, roasting, or air frying.

- Fresh meat and poultry (lean cuts)

- Legumes and beans

- Eggs

- Fresh fruit
  - Bananas
  - Apples
  - Oranges
  - Berries
  - Grapefruits
  - Apricots

- Whole grains
  - Amaranth
  - Barley
  - Buckwheat
  - Brown rice
  - Kamut
  - Quinoa
  - Millet
  - Oats

These grains are intensely delicious and have little to no sodium in them. Like veggies, the key to maintaining their nutrition levels lies in how you prepare them. The trick is to use low-sodium broth or water to boil it.

- Low-fat dairy products
  - Milk
  - Yogurt

We highly recommend plain yogurts because they are naturally low in sodium instead of flavored ones that tend to sneak in salts and sugars. Greek yogurts are great because they are low in sodium and loaded with proteins, making them an excellent option for a healthy heart.

• Herbs and spices

Using herbs and spices make a tremendous difference in your cooking. They add flavor and depth to your food and significantly cut down on the sugar and sodium levels in your food. Don't just eat boring, bland food! Experiment with different vibrant flavors that will take your cooking a notch higher. Reach out for turmeric, mint, sage, cumin, and any other herb you would typically not use.

• Unsalted nuts/seeds

What I love most about nuts is that they offer a crunchy texture and are packed with proteins. According to studies, people who consume nuts regularly have a lower risk of developing heart and heart-related complications. If you can't completely steer clear of salted nuts, try mixing salted and unsalted in a 1:3 ratio. This way, you cut down on the salt intake while enjoying all the nutrients that come along with every bite, like omega-3 fatty acids.

It should be noted that even if something is naturally low in sodium, it might still have added salt or spices that bump up the sodium level. For instance, celery is naturally low in sodium, but adding salt or pepper bumps it up to moderate levels.

When you find low-sodium options at the grocery store, look for "no added salt" labels so that you know exactly what you're getting.

Food List and Sodium Content

Now that you have a good idea of what foods to look for and avoid, here's a curated list of the most common foods and their sodium content. This list is ideal for those trying to watch their sodium intake and looking for meal ideas, but it's also a great reference guide for anyone who wants to know more about the foods they eat daily.

Food	Weight (grams)	Portion	Sodium (milligrams)
Beverages			
Light beer	354	12 fl oz	11
Regular beer, regular	355	12 fl oz	18
Red wine	103	3.5 fl oz	5
White wine	103	3.5 fl oz	5
Unsweetened apple juice (no ascorbic acid)	248	1 cup	7
Club soda	355	12 fl oz	75
Cola	370	12 fl oz	15
Ginger ale	366	12 fl oz	26
Chocolate powder mix	266	1 cup	165
Espresso	60	2 fl oz	8

Brewed coffee	178	6 fl oz	4
Sweetened grapefruit juice (canned)	250	1 cup	5
Raw pink grapefruit juice	247	1 cup	2
Vanilla milkshake	313	11 fl oz	297
Low-fat milk chocolate	250	1 cup	153
Low-fat milk (1% milkfat, vitamin A)	244	1 cup	124
Non-fat or skim milk (vitamin A)	245	1 cup	127
Raw orange juice	248	1 cup	2
Soy milk	245	1 cup	29
Brewed chamomile tea	178	6 fl oz	2
Dairy products and eggs			
Salted butter	14.2	1 tbsp	117
Unsalted butter	14.2	1 tbsp	2
Home-prepared cheese sauce	243	1 cup	1,198
Cheddar cheese	28.35	1 oz	176
Cream cottage cheese	210	1 cup	851
Low-fat cottage cheese (1% milkfat)	226	1 cup	918
Cream cheese	14.5	1 tbsp	43
Feta cheese	28.35	1 oz	316

Half and half cream	15	1 tbsp	6
Cultured sour cream	12	1 tbsp	6
Whipped cream	3	1 tbsp	4
Liquid egg substitute	62.75	1/4 cup	111
Hard-boiled egg	50	1 large	62
Raw egg	44	1 medium	55
Raw egg	50	1 large	63
Soft-serve vanilla yogurt	72	1/2 cup	63
Sweetened condensed milk	306	1 cup	389
Low-fat fruit yogurt (10g protein per 8oz)	227	8-oz container	132
Low-fat plain yogurt (12g protein per 8oz)	227	8-oz container	159
Plain skim milk yogurt (13g protein per 8oz)	227	8-oz container	175
Plain whole milk yogurt (8g protein per 8oz)	227	8-oz container	104
Fats and oils			
Regular margarine (added salt)	14.1	1 tbsp	133
Soft margarine (added salt)	4.7	1 tsp	51

Margarine-like spread (about 40% fat)	4.8	1 tsp	46
Margarine-like spread, (about 60% fat, soybean and palm)	14.4	1 tbsp	143
Olive oil	13.5	1 tbsp	0
Canola oil	14	1 tbsp	0
Corn oil	13.6	1 tbsp	0
Soybean oil	13.6	1 tbsp	0
Sunflower oil (60% and over)	13.6	1 tbsp	0
Salad dressing (mayonnaise or soybean oil, salted)	13.8	1 tbsp	78
Fish and shellfish			
Cooked lobster	85	3 oz	323
Canned shrimp	85.05	3 oz	144
Tuna salad	205	1 cup	824
Canned white tuna	85	3 oz	320
Fried breaded scallops	93	6 large	432
Fruits and fruit juices			
Apples	138	1 apple	0
Canned sweetened applesauce (unsalted)	255	1 cup	8
Avocados	28.35	1 oz	3

Bananas	118	1 banana	1
Sweetened blueberries	230	1 cup	2
Blueberries	145	1 cup	9
Cherries (canned or heavy syrup)	68	10 cherries	0
Frozen desserts, fruit and juice bars	77	1 bar (2.5 fl oz)	3
Pink and red grapefruit	123	1/2 grapefruit	0
White grapefruit	118	1/2 grapefruit	0
Kiwi fruit	76	1 medium	4
Lemon juice (canned or bottled)	15.2	1 tbsp	3
Fresh lemon juice	47	juice of 1 lemon	0
Cantaloupe	69	1/8 melon	6
Honeydew	170	1 cup	17
Nectarines	136	1 nectarine	0
Canned ripe olives	22	5 large	192
Oranges	131	1 orange	0
Papayas	140	1 cup	4

Canned peaches (solids and liquids)	248	1 cup	10
Peaches	98	1 peach	0
Pears	166	1 pear	0
Canned pineapple (solids and liquids)	249	1 cup	2
Pineapple	155	1 cup	2
Plantains	179	1 medium	7
Plums	66	1 plum	0
Uncooked dried prunes	42	5 prunes	2
Boiled pumpkin (unsalted)	245	1 cup	2
Seedless raisins	145	1 cup	17
Frozen and sweetened raspberries	250	1 cup	3
Raspberries	123	1 cup	0
Fruit leather	28.35	1 oz	114
Frozen and sweetened strawberries	255	1 cup	8
Strawberries	166	1 cup	2
Watermelon	152	1 cup	3
Grain products			
Plain bagels	71	3-1/2" bagel	379
Homemade biscuits	60	2-1/2" biscuit	348

Bread stuffing	100	1/2 cup	543
Bread (mixed-grain, whole-grain, or 7-grain)	26	1 slice	127
Oatmeal bread	27	1 slice	162
Rye bread	32	1 slice	211
Toasted rye bread	24	1 slice	174
Whole-wheat bread	28	1 slice	148
Cereals (wheat germ, toasted, and plain)	7.1	1 tbsp	0
Cereals (wheat, puffed, and fortified)	12	1 cup	0
Cheese crackers	10	10 crackers	100
Plain melba toast	20	4 pieces	166
Saltines (includes oyster, soda, soup)	12	4 crackers	156
Wheat crackers	8	4 crackers	64
Whole-wheat crackers	16	4 crackers	105
Butter croissants	57	1 croissant	424
Seasoned croutons	40	1 cup	495
English muffins and sourdough	52	1 muffin	262
Egg noodles	160	1 cup	11

Spinach egg noodles	160	1 cup	19
Pancakes	38	1 pancake	192
Pasta with meatballs in tomato sauce	252	1 cup	1,053
Brown, long-grain rice	195	1 cup	10
White, long-grain rice	185	1 cup	9
Dinner rolls	28	1 roll	146
Hamburger or hot dog rolls	43	1 roll	241
Barbecue-flavored chips (corn base)	28.35	1 oz	216
Cheese-flavored puffs or twists (corn base)	28.35	1 oz	298
Granola bars	28.35	1 bar	83
Ready-to-heat waffles (includes buttermilk)	33	1 waffle	260
Plain homemade waffles	75	1 waffle	383
All-purpose wheat flour	125	1 cup	1,588
Wild rice	164	1 cup	5
Legumes, nuts, and seeds			
Plain or vegetarian beans	254	1 cup	1,008

Baked or canned beans with pork and tomato sauce	253	1 cup	1,113
Red kidney beans	256	1 cup	873
Navy beans (unsalted)	182	1 cup	2
Chickpeas (garbanzo beans, Bengal gram)	240	1 cup	718
unsalted chickpeas (garbanzo beans, Bengal gram)	164	1 cup	11
Hummus	14	1 tbsp	53
Lentils (unsalted salt)	198	1 cup	4
Lima beans	241	1 cup	810
Almonds	28.35	1 oz (24 nuts)	0
Dry and roasted cashew nuts (with added salt)	28.35	1 oz	181
Dried coconut meat	93	1 cup	244
Dry and roasted mixed nuts with peanuts (with added salt)	28.35	1 oz	190
Pecans	28.35	1 oz (20 halves)	0
English walnut	28.35	1 oz (14 halves)	1
Chunky peanut butter (salted)	16	1 tbsp	78

Smooth peanut butter (salted)	16	1 tbsp	75
All types dry-roasted peanuts (salted)	28.35	1 oz (approx 28)	230
All types dry-roasted peanuts (unsalted)	28.35	1 oz (approx 28)	2
Refried canned beans	252	1 cup	753
Roasted pumpkin and squash seed kernels (salted)	28.35	1 oz (142 seeds)	163
Sesame butter, tahini	15	1 tbsp	17
Dry roasted sunflower seed kernels (salted)	32	1/4 cup	250
Soy milk	245	1 cup	29
Tofu, firm, prepared with calcium sulfate and magnesium chloride (nigari)	81	1/4 block	6
Soft tofu	120	1 piece	10
Meat, poultry, and related products			
Canned beef stew	232	1 cup	947
Dried cured beef	28.35	1 oz	984
Extra lean ground beef	85	3 oz	60
Top sirloin beef (1/4" fat)	85	3 oz	56

Beef and pork bologna	56.7	2 slices	578
Frozen chicken pot pie	217	1 small pie	857
Chicken breast (skinless)	86	1/2 breast	64
Chicken drumstick (skinless)	44	1 drumstick	42
Chicken wing	49	1 wing	157
Beef frankfurter	45	1 frank	462
Chicken frankfurter	45	1 frank	617
Extra lean ham (about 5% fat)	56.7	2 slices	810
Frozen beef macaroni	240	1 package	444
Choice lamb loin (1/4" fat)	85	3 oz	71
Pork sausage	26	2 links	336
Pork sausage	27	1 patty	349
Cured bacon	19	3 medium slices	303
Canadian-style bacon	46.5	2 slices	719
Cured ham	85	3 oz	1,128
Leg ham	85	3 oz	54
Center loin or chops,	85	3 oz	51

Center rib loin	85	3 oz	40
Beef and pork salami	56.7	2 slices	604
Beef jerky	19.8	1 large piece	438
Mixed dishes and fast foods			
Biscuit with egg and sausage	180	1 biscuit	1,141
Chili con carne with beans	222	1 cup	1,032
Pizza with cheese	63	1 slice	336
Pizza with cheese, meat, and vegetables	79	1 slice	382
Burritos with beans and meat	115.5	1 burrito	668
Cheeseburger with condiments and vegetables	219	1 sandwich	1,108
Cheeseburger, double patty and a bun	160	1 sandwich	891
Plain cheeseburger, double patty	155	1 sandwich	636
Plain chicken filet sandwich	182	1 sandwich	957
Breaded boneless chicken	106	6 pieces	513
Chili con carne	253	1 cup	1,007
Coleslaw	99	3/4 cup	267

Croissants with egg, cheese, and bacon	129	1 croissant	889
English muffins with egg, cheese, and Canadian bacon	137	1 muffin	729
Fish sandwich, with tartar sauce and cheese	183	1 sandwich	939
Plain hot dogs	98	1 sandwich	670
Soft-serve vanilla ice milk with cone	103	1 cone	92
Nachos with cheese	113	6-8 nachos	816
Pancakes with butter and syrup	232	2 pancakes	1,104
French fries (fried in vegetable oil)	85	1 small	168
French fries (fried in vegetable oil)	169	1 large	335
Beef macaroni	240	1 package	444
Low-fat homestyle waffles	35	1 waffle	155
Cheeseburger with bacon and condiments	195	1 sandwich	1,043
Plain cheeseburger	102	1 sandwich	500

Hamburger with condiments and vegetables	218	1 sandwich	824
Soups, sauces, and gravies			
Canned beef gravy	58.25	1/4 cup	326
Canned turkey gravy	59.6	1/4 cup	344
Barbecue sauce	15.75	1 tbsp	128
Ready-to-serve cheese sauce	63	1/4 cup	522
Spaghetti or marinara sauce	250	1 cup	1,030
Salsa sauce	16	1 tbsp	69
Teriyaki sauce	18	1 tbsp	690
Canned bean with pork soup	253	1 cup	951
Canned tomato soup	244	1 cup	695
Canned vegetable soup	241	1 cup	822
Pancake syrups	20	1 tbsp	17
Reduced-calorie pancake syrup	15	1 tbsp	30
Canned tomato paste paste (unsalted)	262	1 cup	231
Canned tomato sauce	245	1 cup	1,482
Sugars and sweets			
Angel food cake	28	1 piece	210

Dry mix angel food cake	50	1 piece	255
Chocolate cake	95	1 piece	299
Gingerbread cake	74	1 piece	242
Fat-free pound cake	28	1 slice	95
White cake with coconut frosting	112	1 piece	318
White cake	74	1 piece	242
Gumdrops, starch jelly	74	10 worms	33
Hard candies	6	1 piece	2
Chocolate chip cookie	10	1 cookie	32
Low-fat chocolate chip cookies	10	1 cookie	38
Fig bars	16	1 cookie	56
Molasses	15	1 cookie, medium	69
Peanut butter cookies	20	1 cookie	104
Vanilla sandwich cookie with cream filling	15	1 cookie	52
Fruit and juice bars	77	1 bar (2.5 fl oz)	3
Vanilla ice cream	66	1/2 cup	53
Orange sherbet	74	1/2 cup	34

Soft-serve vanilla yogurt	72	1/2 cup	63
Jams and preserves	20	1 tbsp	6
Blackstrap molasses	20	1 tbsp	11
Pie crust	180	1 pie shell	976
Apple pie	155	1 piece	327
Blueberry pie	147	1 piece	272
Cherry pie	180	1 piece	344
Fried fruit pie	128	1 pie	479
Lemon meringue pie	127	1 piece	307
Pumpkin pie	155	1 piece	349
Plain granola bars	28.35	1 bar	83
Vegetables and vegetable products			
Asparagus	60	4 spears	7
Frozen asparagus (unsalted)	180	1 cup	7
Canned green beans	135	1 cup	354
Green beans (unsalted)	125	1 cup	4
Beet greens (unsalted)	144	1 cup	347
Canned beets	170	1 cup	330
Beets	170	1 cup	131

Cooked broccoli (unsalted)	156	1 cup	41
Broccoli	88	1 cup	24
Brussels sprouts (unsalted)	156	1 cup	33
Frozen brussels sprouts (unsalted)	155	1 cup	36
Cabbage	70	1 cup	13
Cooked carrots (unsalted)	156	1 cup	103
Carrots	110	1 cup	39
Frozen cauliflower (unsalted)	180	1 cup	32
Cauliflower	100	1 cup	30
Celery	120	1 cup	104
Home-prepared coleslaw	120	1 cup	28
Cream-style sweet corn	256	1 cup	730
Vacuum pack sweet corn	210	1 cup	571
Cooked sweet corn (unsalted)	77	1 ear	13
Frozen sweet corn (unsalted)	164	1 cup	8
Peeled cucumber	119	1 cup	2
Cucumber	104	1 cup	2
Dandelion greens (unsalted)	105	1 cup	46
Eggplant (unsalted)	99	1 cup	3

Romaine lettuce	56	1 cup	4
Onion rings	60	10 rings	225
Onions	160	1 cup	5
Onion spring or scallions (with tops and bulb)	15	1 whole	2
Edible-pod (unsalted)	160	1 cup	6
Home-prepared potato pancakes	76	1 pancake	386
Potato puffs	79	10 puffs	589
Home-prepared potato salad	250	1 cup	1,323
Au gratin potatoes	245	1 cup	1,061
Baked potatoes (unsalted)	156	1 potato	8
Miscellaneous items			
Ketchup	15	1 tbsp	178
Baking powder (with sodium aluminum sulfate)	4.6	1 tsp	488
Baking powder (with straight phosphate)	4.6	1 tsp	363
Baking powder (with low-sodium)	5	1 tsp	5
Baking soda	4.6	1 tsp	1,259
Active dry baker's yeast	7	1 pkg	4

Miso	68.75	1 cup	2,507
Yellow mustard	5	1 tsp or 1 packet	56
Sweet pickle relish	15	1 tbsp	122
Dill cucumber	65	1 pickle	833
Canned pimento	12	1 tbsp	2
Table salt	6	1 tsp	2,325
Shoyu	16	1 tbsp	914
Cider vinegar	15	1 tbsp	0
Tap water	237	8 fl oz	7

Sample Low Sodium Recipes

Arugula and Mushroom Salad

Ingredients:
- 5 oz. arugula washed
- 1 lb. fresh mushrooms
- 1/4 tsp. shoyu
- 1/2 red onion
- 1 tbsp. olive oil
- 1 tbsp. mirin

For tofu cheese:
- 1/8 cup umeboshi vinegar
- 1/2 firm tofu

Instructions:
1. In a bowl, add the rinsed tofu. Crumble and pour in vinegar.
2. In a separate bowl add shoyu, red onions, salt, olive oil, and mirin. 3. Mix to combine.
4. Add in the arugula and toss to combine with the dressing.
5. Serve and enjoy.

Asian Zucchini Salad

Ingredients:
- 1 medium zucchini, sliced thinly into spirals
- 1/3 cup rice vinegar
- 3/4 cup avocado oil
- 1 cup sunflower seeds, shells removed
- 1 lb. cabbage, shredded
- 1 tsp. stevia drops
- 1 cup almonds, sliced

Instructions:
1. Cut the zucchini spirals into smaller parts. Set aside.
2. Put almonds, sunflower seeds, and cabbage in a large bowl. Combine the ingredients well.
4. Add zucchini to the mixture.
5. In a small bowl, mix vinegar, stevia, and oil using a whisk or fork.
6. Pour vinegar mixture all over the zucchini mixture. Toss well. Make sure everything is covered with the dressing.
7. Refrigerate for 2 hours before serving.

Crispy Brussels Sprouts

Ingredients:
- 2 cups Brussels sprouts
- 1 tbsp. olive oil
- 1 tbsp. balsamic vinegar

Instructions:
1. Put all the ingredients in a bowl and toss them well.
2. Put the Brussels in the air fryer basket and cook for 8 minutes at 400°F. Check the progress after 5 minutes.
3. Serve hot and enjoy the crispy Brussel sprouts.

Grenade Salad

Ingredients:
- 4 cups arugula
- 1 large avocado
- 1/2 cup sliced fennel
- 1/2 cup sliced Anjou pears
- 1/4 cup pomegranate seeds

Instructions:
1. Mix all the ingredients except for the pomegranate seeds.
2. After mixing well, add the seeds. Mix again.
3. Serve with any type of desired dressing.

Kale Salad with Strawberry & Almonds

Ingredients:
- 1 bunch of kale
- 1/2 cup sliced strawberries
- 1/4 cup sliced almonds
- 1 lemon pulp juice
- 1/8 tsp. salt
- 1/8 tsp. black pepper
- 1 tbsp. agave
- 2 tbsp. of olive oil

Instructions:
1. Rip kale into small pieces and massage with hands until tender.
2. Put it in a bowl. Add almonds and strawberries.
3. To create a dressing, mix lemon juice with olive oil, salt, pepper, and agave, and then pour it over the salad.
4. Serve immediately.

Baked Potato Delight

Ingredients:
- 1 medium russet potato, clean and patted dry
- olive oil

Instructions:
1. Preheat your air fryer to 400°F.
2. Poke holes on both sides of each potato with a fork.
3. Drizzle some olive oil.
4. Place the potatoes in a layer over the air fryer basket and cook them for around 40 minutes.
5. Once the potatoes are baked, slice them using a fork.
6. Add cheese or ketchup as toppings.
7. Serve and enjoy them while hot.

Prosciutto-Roast Beef Tenderloin

Ingredients:
- 4-lb. whole beef tenderloin, tail removed
- 1 tbsp. garlic, finely chopped or crushed
- 1 tbsp. olive oil
- 1/4 tsp. ground black pepper
- 1 tsp. fresh parsley, chopped
- 4 oz. prosciutto, deli-sliced

Instructions:
1. Preheat the oven to 425°F.
2. Place the tenderloin on a chopping board.
3. In a bowl, combine the olive oil, garlic, pepper, and parsley. Rub the garlic mix over the tenderloin.
4. Wrap the tenderloin gently with overlapping prosciutto ribbons until covered. On a roasting pan or cookie sheet, place the tenderloin.
5. Roast until desired doneness is achieved. Roast for 26 to 28 minutes for rare, 30 minutes for medium-rare, and 35 to 40 minutes for well-done.
6. Remove from the oven and allow to rest for 10 minutes before slicing the tenderloin.
7. Serve either cold or warm.

Chicken Breast with Parmesan Crust

Ingredients:
- 1 lb. or 3 pcs. chicken breasts, cut horizontally in halves
- 1 tsp. any Italian seasoning
- 1/2 tsp. garlic powder
- black pepper
- 1 cup grated parmesan cheese
- 1/2 cup panko bread crumbs
- 2 tbsp. olive oil
- 2 large eggs

Instructions:
1. Season the chicken breasts with pepper, garlic powder, and Italian spices. Set them aside.
2. In a shallow bowl, add parmesan cheese along with panko bread crumbs. Mix them well.
3. In another bowl, add eggs and whisk them together.
4. Dip the chicken breasts into the beaten egg and then into the cheese mixture. Repeat the process with all the cutlets.
5. Pour some olive oil into a heavy-duty skillet and heat.
6. Put the chicken breasts in a single layer. Cook each side for 6 minutes or until the sides turn golden. Repeat the process with the remaining chicken breasts.
7. Serve them hot with tomato ketchup or any of your favorite dips.

Crispy Shrimp in Coconut

Ingredients:
- 20 pcs. large shrimps, patted dry with paper towels
- 2 pcs. eggs, beaten
- 1/2 cup shredded coconut
- 1/2 cup all-purpose flour
- 1/4 cup panko bread crumbs
- 1/4 tsp. black pepper
- cooking spray

Instructions:
1. Preheat the air fryer to 400°F.
2. In a bowl, add panko bread crumbs along with shredded coconut and pepper. Mix them well.
3. Dip shrimps in the egg mixture and then press them into the panko-coconut mixture. Make sure to coat all sides.
4. Place the shrimps in a single layer inside the air fryer basket.
5. Bake them for 5 minutes.
6. Serve them hot.

<u>Crunchy Popcorn Chicken</u>

Ingredients:
- 1 lb. skinless chicken cubes
- 1/2 cup cornstarch
- 1/2 tsp. onion powder
- 1/2 tsp. garlic powder
- 1 cup unsweetened coconut milk
- 1/2 tsp. paprika
- 3 cups crushed cornflakes
- 1/4 tsp. cayenne pepper
- 1/4 tsp. black pepper
- 1 tsp. pickle juice

Instructions:
1. Pour the cornstarch onto a plate and set aside.
2. In a bowl, mix the coconut milk and pickle juice.
3. Take a plastic bag and add cornflakes along with the spices. Crush the flakes and pour them onto a plate.
4. Coat the chicken cubes with cornstarch and then dip them into the coconut milk. Now, roll them over the flake crumbs. Repeat the process with all the chicken cubes.
5. Take out the air fryer basket and lightly coat it with cooking spray. Place the chicken cubes in a single layer.
6. Bake the cubes at 400°F for 10 minutes.
7. Once they turn golden, take them out.
8. Serve hot.

Steak and Lime

Ingredients:
- 1 flank steak
- 1 lime
- 2 cloves garlic, pressed
- 2 tbsp. parsley
- 2 tbsp. avocado oil
- coarse salt

Instructions:
1. Mix oil with pressed garlic, parsley, and the juice of half a lime.
2. Pour mixture over both sides of flank steak and sprinkle salt as well.
3. Let marinate for 30 minutes.
4. Grill or bake the steak, whichever you prefer.
5. Serve and enjoy while warm.

Raspberry Blueberry Smoothie

Ingredients:
- 1 cup fresh raspberries, frozen
- 1 cup wild blueberries, frozen
- 1 tbsp. flaxseed, freshly ground
- 3/4 cup rice milk
- 3/4 cup ice, crushed

Instructions:
1. Put all the ingredients in the food processor.
2. Blend until the texture has become smooth.
3. Pour into the preferred container.
4. Serve immediately.

Breakfast Smoothie

Ingredients:
- 1 ripe banana, frozen
- 1 cup strawberries, frozen
- 1/2 cup pomegranate arils, frozen or fresh
- 4 cups leafy green vegetable, fresh or lightly steamed
- 1/2 cup broccoli florets, frozen
- 10 mint leaves, fresh
- 1 lime, juiced
- fresh ginger, about an inch
- 1/4 cup hemp seeds
- 3 cups filtered water
- 2 tbsp. Flax meal
- 2 tbsp. cocoa powder

Instructions:
1. Put hemp seeds and water into a high-speed blender.
2. Add the banana, strawberries, and pomegranate arils.
3. Add the leafy green vegetable, broccoli, mint, lime juice, ginger, flax meal, and cocoa powder.
4. Cover the blender with its lid.
5. Turn on the blender for about 45 seconds, or until the texture of the smoothie has become smooth.
6. Pour into the preferred container.
7. Serve and enjoy.

Healthy Green Smoothie

Ingredients:
- 1 cup fresh spinach
- 1/2 tsp. mint extract or to taste
- Optional: 1/4 tsp. peppermint liquid Stevia

Instructions:
1. Gather the ingredients.
2. Add them to a high-powered blender.
3. Turn on the blender.
4. Add them to the glass and freeze for 5 minutes.
5. Serve and enjoy.

Conclusion

It is no secret that sodium is an important electrolyte in the body that plays a key role in maintaining a healthy fluid balance, nerve impulse transmission, and muscle contraction.

However, while sodium does a lot of good to our bodies, consuming it in excess can cause many health problems. Most people still consume more sodium than is required, which increases its concentration in the bloodstream. This poses several health risks like heart and heart-related problems.

This is why it is important to moderate your sodium intake!

By following the tips, we have discussed in this guide; you are sure to lower your sodium intake to acceptable limits. The trick is to consume a low-sodium diet, which goes a long way in improving blood pressure, lowering chronic kidney diseases, and improving the overall quality of life.

Always go for fresh fruits and veggies, whole grains foods, and low-fat dairy products. Additionally, increase your Potassium intake, drink plenty of water, increase your physical activity, and control your salt intake.

Now you know what to do. So, what are you still waiting for?

It's time to ditch those high-sodium foods for healthier low-sodium foods that are good for you.

References

Aburto, N. J., Ziolkovska, A., Hooper, L., Elliott, P., Cappuccio, F. P., & Meerpohl, J. J. (2013). Effect of lower sodium intake on health: systematic review and meta-analyses. Bmj, 346, f1326.

Calliope, S. R., & Samman, N. C. (2020). Sodium content in commonly consumed foods and its contribution to the daily intake. Nutrients, 12(1), 34.

CDC. (2022, August 19). Sodium and health. Centers for Disease Control and Prevention. https://www.cdc.gov/salt/index.htm.

Doyle, M. E., & Glass, K. A. (2010). Sodium reduction and its effect on food safety, food quality, and human health. Comprehensive reviews in food science and food safety, 9(1), 44-56.

Farquhar, W. B., Edwards, D. G., Jurkovitz, C. T., & Weintraub, W. S. (2015). Dietary sodium and health: more than just blood pressure. Journal of the American College of Cardiology, 65(10), 1042-1050.

How to track your sodium. (n.d.). Www.Heart.Org. Retrieved September 1, 2022, from https://www.heart.org/en/healthy-living/healthy-eating/eat-smart/sodium/how-to-track-your-sodium.

Kirkpatrick, S. I., Raffoul, A., Lee, K. M., & Jones, A. C. (2019). Top dietary sources of energy, sodium, sugars, and saturated fats among Canadians: Insights from the 2015 Canadian Community Health Survey. Applied Physiology, Nutrition, and Metabolism, 44(6), 650-658.

Mente, A., O'Donnell, M., & Yusuf, S. (2021). Sodium intake and health: What should we recommend based on the current evidence? Nutrients, 13(9), 3232.

Mitchell, H. (2016). Developing food products for consumers with low sodium/salt requirements. In Developing food products for consumers with specific dietary needs (pp. 81-105). Woodhead Publishing.

Safe, I. L. Sodium Content of Your Food. Bulletin #4059. (extension.umaine.edu).

Salt reduction. (n.d.). Retrieved September 1, 2022, from https://www.who.int/news-room/fact-sheets/detail/salt-reduction.

CPSIA information can be obtained
at www.ICGtesting.com
Printed in the USA
BVHW051744060323
659810BV00006B/142

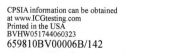

9 781088 082621